HELLO NEW YOU

EAT BETTER, DRINK LESS, EXERCISE MORE

KATHERINE BEBO

summersdale

An Hachette UK Company
www.hachette.co.uk

Summersdale Publishers Ltd
Part of Octopus Publishing Group Limited
Carmelite House
50 Victoria Embankment
LONDON
EC4Y 0DZ
UK

www.summersdale.com

Printed and bound in the Czech Republic

ISBN: 978-1-78685-759-0

Substantial discounts on bulk quantities of Summersdale books are available to corporations, professional associations and other organisations. For details contact general enquiries by telephone: +44 (0) 1243 771107 or email: enquiries@summersdale.com

For Mum. I always eat better when you're around.

CONTENTS

INTRODUCTION:
THE GREATEST WEALTH
IS HEALTH

To keep the body in good health is a duty... otherwise we shall not be able to keep our mind strong and clear.

BUDDHA

Eat better... Drink less... Exercise more... Sounds simple enough. But as with many things in life – like vowing not to hit the snooze button, updating your CV, or getting round to defrosting your freezer – sometimes things are easier said than done. Often, we need a little helping hand to transform our good intentions into reality. Which is where this book comes in. Whether it's matching your workout to your mood or choosing foods that will boost your sex life, it's chock-full of tips, advice and encouragement to help you on your journey to a happier, healthier you. Remember, if you're good to your body, your body will be good to you.

PART 1
EAT BETTER

One cannot think well, love well, sleep well, if one has not dined well.

Virginia Woolf

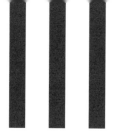

A HELPING HAND

Not sure how much of each food type you should be eating to be healthy and stay in shape? Your hand is a perfectly good portion guide for the main meal of your day:

- Protein: the size of your palm.
- Vegetables: the size of your outstretched hand.
- Carbs and fruit: the size of your closed fist.
- Cooking fats like butter and oil: the size of one fingertip.
- Nuts, cheese and other high-fat foods: the size of your thumb.

BRING ON THE SUBSTITUTES

Allergies... Religion... Intolerance... Veganism... Plain fussiness... There are many reasons why people don't eat certain foods. But eliminating a whole food group means you're missing out on all the good stuff it brings, and this can have an adverse effect on your health if you don't have a balanced diet. These alternatives will help your body stay in tip-top condition:

- If you don't eat **MEAT**, try soya products, pulses, eggs, beans, peas, lentils, crab and Brazil nuts for a protein kick.
- If you don't eat **FISH**, try flaxseeds, pumpkin seeds, sunflower seeds, olives and offal for a dose of omega-3 fatty acids.
- If you don't eat **DAIRY**, try fortified soya milk, soya yogurt, tofu, almonds, pulses, sardines and green vegetables like broccoli for your all-important calcium.
- If you don't eat **WHEAT**, try oats, brown rice and other unrefined grains for fibre.

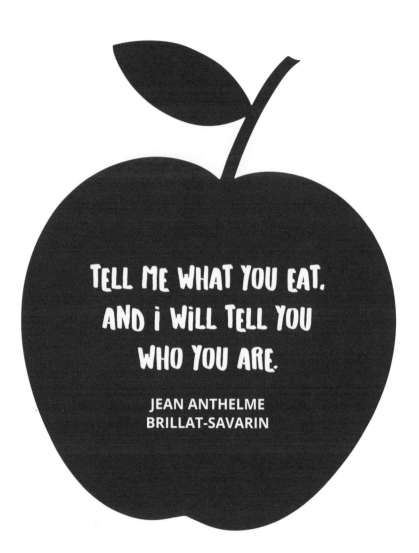

TELL ME WHAT YOU EAT,
AND I WILL TELL YOU
WHO YOU ARE.

JEAN ANTHELME
BRILLAT-SAVARIN

DON'T CUT CARBS COMPLETELY

It's a common misconception that carbohydrates are fattening when, in fact, they contain the same amount of calories per gram (four) as protein. Carbs are essential to the body for energy, and it's advisable never to cut them out of your diet completely.

AT A LOSS

A calorie deficit is when you burn more calories than you consume, which forces the body to use non-food sources of energy – typically body fat. If you want to lose weight, a calorie deficit is the only way you're going to do it.

SEX UP YOUR DIET

These fruits and vegetables will boost your sex life, meaning you'll burn calories and inspire healthy weight loss. Yes, (yes, yes) really!

BANANAS – As they contain the enzyme bromelain, bananas are believed to increase libido and reverse impotence in men.

FIGS – These sweet, sticky fruits are bursting with amino acids, which invigorate your sex drive and raise sexual stamina.

POMEGRANATES – Pomegranate juice helps the body to produce nitric oxide, which opens blood vessels to increase blood flow. This is helpful to men who experience impotence.

ASPARAGUS – This spring vegetable is rich in vitamin E, which stimulates the production of testosterone – a hormone crucial for a great sex life for both men and women.

GARLIC – Garlic contains allicin – the pungent compound responsible for the bulb's strong smell – which increases blood flow. It is thought that increased blood flow can boost sexual desire and aid erectile dysfunction. If the pong of garlic leaves you feeling anything but sexy, try garlic capsules instead.

MACA – This root vegetable contains p-methoxybenzyl isothiocyanate, which has aphrodisiac properties. For men, it is believed to improve sperm count and combat impotence; for women, it perks up a low sex drive.

AVOCADOS – High in vitamin B6 and potassium, avocados raise hormone production and help to regulate the thyroid gland, which can boost libido.

PUMPKIN SEEDS – These are packed with zinc, which is key for men's testosterone production. A zinc deficiency can also zap a woman's sex drive completely.

GO DARK

Dark-coloured fruits and vegetables – like blueberries, leafy greens, prunes and pomegranates – are one of the best sources of antioxidant phytochemicals, which fight disease and boost immunity. So if you say 'pah' to plums or 'bleugh' to blackberries, you may be more susceptible to illness.

HEALTH IS NOT ABOUT THE WEIGHT YOU LOSE, BUT ABOUT THE LIFE YOU GAIN.

MAKE YOUR TASTE BUDS POP

Many people don't realize that popcorn is actually good for you. Popcorn is a wholegrain, and it's advisable to eat three servings of wholegrains every day (just not all popcorn!) for a healthy gut. Obviously, popcorn becomes less healthy if you add sugar, butter or salt. Instead, try sprinkling cinnamon or paprika over it.

POPCORN FOR
BREAKFAST! WHY NOT?
IT'S A GRAIN. IT'S
LIKE GRITS. BUT WITH
HIGH SELF-ESTEEM.

James Patterson

DON'T MINDLESSLY MUNCH

Do you often intend to only eat a handful of nibbles but before you know it – oh dear – the entire 'sharing' bag is gone? If so, you may be a 'mindless eater'. You'll often eat when distracted, like when you're watching TV. To combat your gratuitous gorging, try to eat with no distractions so you can concentrate on identifying when you're full. Also, keep a food record so you're aware of what you're putting in your mouth. Knowing you're going to be writing down your food intake will make you think twice about those extra squares of chocolate. Another way to be mindful when you're snacking is to portion out your food. Instead of eating straight from the bag, empty a serving into a bowl and put the bag away. When they're gone, they're gone.

LIVIN' LA VEGAN LOCA

There's often a mistaken belief that vegans can't conceivably be healthy. Where do they get their nutrients from? What do they actually eat? Surely just hummus, right? Tsk! Vegans can indeed be very healthy and eat a host of delicious foods. They often take in more nutrients than their non-vegan counterparts. Spinach and kale, for example, contain more iron per gram than beef, and better quality protein comes from beans or soy products than from meat.

EAT LIFE IN THE SLOW LANE

Fast-release carbs like bread and cereal create a sharp rise and fall in blood sugar levels, which leads to cravings for sugary foods. On the other hand, slow-release carbs with a low glycaemic index (GI) will keep your blood sugar levels, er, level. Go for seeds, nuts, legumes, peas and wholegrains.

EAT LEAN, CLEAN, FRESH AND GREEN.

A healthy outside starts from the inside.

Robert Urich

PRETTY COOL STUFF

Cooled pasta is less fattening than just-cooked pasta, and reheated pasta is less fattening still. Why? The structure of the pasta gets converted to 'resistant starch' while cooling, and an even more resistant starch when reheated. The body can't break down or absorb this and so treats resistant starch more like fibre than a carbohydrate. Fibre helps with digestive function, and balances blood sugar levels, so you'll absorb fewer calories and won't experience the rise and fall in blood glucose that occurs when you gorge on carbohydrates (which can make you feel hungry again soon after you've eaten). With cooled pasta, you'll feel satisfied and will have fewer cravings. The same is true for rice and potatoes – eaten cold, they contain more resistant starch.

NOTHING TO SNIFF AT

Vitamins A, C, D and E, plus iron and zinc, are the most important nutrients to support your immune system. Incorporating plenty of oranges, nuts, seeds and leafy green vegetables into your diet will help keep the sniffles at bay. As will eating hearty soups containing lentils and beans.

How to lose weight: turn your head to the left, turn your head to the right. Repeat this exercise whenever you are offered chocolate cake.

REFUSE TO FEED GREED

If you want to reduce
your appetite, try these tips:

- Serve yourself a portion, then put the leftovers out of sight.
- Use a smaller plate or bowl.
- Don't ever eat while standing in front of the fridge.

LiFE EXPECTANCY WOULD GROW BY LEAPS AND BOUNDS iF GREEN VEGETABLES SMELLED AS GOOD AS BACON.

DOUG LARSON

THE FRIDGE IS A CLEAR EXAMPLE THAT WHAT MATTERS IS ON THE INSIDE.

GO SLOW

The feeling of fullness takes about
20 minutes to reach your brain.
To avoid overeating, munch slowly to
allow your brain to get the message.
Taking your time with food will
also increase your enjoyment
of the flavours.

FAT IS YOUR FRIEND

Many people avoid fat when they are trying to eat healthily. But they shouldn't. It can help with weight management. Unsaturated fat, or 'good fat', encourages a healthy heart and can help keep you trim by boosting metabolic health, keeping you fuller for longer and building muscle. Fat is essential in the diet for a number of reasons:

- Fat aids the absorption of essential fatty acids and fat-soluble vitamins. You will absorb more nutrients from a salad served with a dressing than from one without.

- The digestive process is assisted by fat as it helps the body to absorb vitamins A, D and E. These vitamins are fat-soluble, which means they can only be absorbed with the help of fats.

- Fat helps with cognitive function by increasing the production of the neurotransmitter acetylcholine, which is vital for memory, reasoning and concentration.

- Fatty acids can boost serotonin levels in the brain, improving attitude, mood and motivation, and reducing anxiety.

- Fat helps to improve the condition of skin, hair and nails.

Unsaturated fat can be found in avocados, fish, nuts, seeds, olive oil and leafy vegetables.

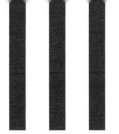

PUSH THE BLOAT OUT

To reduce bloating, drink lots of water. We should guzzle around 1.2 litres (42 fl oz) a day to reduce dehydration and, in turn, water retention and constipation. Probiotic foods that contain 'good bacteria' – like live yogurt – will also help to beat the bloat. As will wholegrains, fruit, nuts, seeds and leafy green veg.

YOU ARE WHAT YOU EAT, SO DON'T BE FAST, CHEAP, EASY OR FAKE.

ACID TRIP

Wrinkles... Dull skin... Aches
and pains... Ugh! Avoiding too much
acidity in foods is important if you don't
want to prematurely age your body
and face. Junk food is a major culprit
here, as is sugar, fried or processed
food, and white-flour products such
as pasta and bread. Balance
is your buddy!

YOUR DIET IS A BANK ACCOUNT.
GOOD FOOD CHOICES ARE
GOOD INVESTMENTS.

BETHENNY FRANKEL

FEED YOUR THYROID

Your thyroid, located at the front of your neck, produces and stores hormones that affect the function of almost every organ in your body. Problems with your thyroid can lead to weight gain, pale skin, fatigue, brittle nails, hair loss, mood swings, depression and headaches. Give your thyroid a kick up the backside by eating kelp because it is high in iodine, drinking herbal teas (such as chamomile or parsley), and increasing vitamins A and D in your diet. Try liver pâté, cheese and eggs for vitamin A, and oily fish, egg yolks and red meat for vitamin D.

REST ASSURED

Can't sleep? Tossing and turning in the middle of the night is no fun at all, but maintaining a healthy weight and eating a varied diet can help you catch the zzzs you need. Some foods will increase your production of melatonin – the hormone that helps you sleep. Try almonds, lettuce, oats, potatoes and turkey (post-Christmas-dinner snooze, anyone?). Bananas can also work wonders in helping you nod off and have been called 'nature's sleeping pill'. The magnesium and potassium they contain will relax muscles and nerves, and the body will be encouraged to produce serotonin, a chemical in your brain that affects mood and will help you feel more chilled out. Drinking chamomile tea or hot milk before bed may also help you fall into a restful slumber. Night, night...

EAT MORE COLOURS.

ALL NIGHT LONG

If you've got a big night out planned and are worried about flagging, eat complex carbs like brown rice at dinnertime. They'll provide slow-release energy to see you into the small hours.

I really regret eating healthily today.

No One Ever

YOU'RE NOT RESPONSIBLE FOR EVERYTHING THAT HAPPENS TO YOU IN LIFE, BUT YOU ARE RESPONSIBLE FOR EVERYTHING YOU PUT IN YOUR BODY.

TAKE GLUTTONY OFF THE MENU

Before going out to a restaurant, look at the menu online first, if possible. That way, you can research the nutritional information before you dine so that you make healthy choices. If you don't want to overindulge, aim to choose a healthy option from the menu. You could, perhaps, opt for a pasta dish with a tomato-based sauce rather than the creamy carbonara, and if you're having a salad, empty the dressing into a dish, then dip your empty fork into it before you spear your lettuce. All the taste, fewer calories.

YOUNG AT HEART
[AND MIND, AND BODY]

To keep your body and mind young, and help slow the ageing process, eat an antioxidant-rich diet. Antioxidants are compounds in food that stop or delay damage to cells by removing waste products before they can do any harm. These foods will slow that ticking clock:

BLUEBERRIES
These blue beauties can help prevent oxidative damage to the nerves in the brain, keeping your memory sharper for longer.

CHILLI PEPPERS
The vitamin C in these hotties can maintain collagen in the skin, which helps it to keep its elasticity.

OILY FISH
There's a correlation between eating food rich in omega-3 and the decreased onset of brain diseases such as dementia. Tuck into oily fish such as mackerel, trout, salmon, sardines and fresh tuna two to three times a week.

WATERCRESS
Packed with vitamins, minerals and phytonutrients, watercress is amazing for the skin – and can help to reduce fine lines and wrinkles.

BEEF and CHICKEN
Including a decent amount of protein in our diet will slow the process of muscle-mass reduction as we age. Beef and chicken also contain coenzyme Q10, which is used to create energy for cell renewal. If you don't eat meat, lentils are a great source of protein.

LEAFY GREEN VEGETABLES
Osteoporosis – brittle bones – becomes more common as we get older. Calcium is crucial to help keep bones strong and dense. Spinach, cabbage and kale will help, as will drinking plenty of milk or calcium-fortified non-dairy alternatives.

DON'T BE LISTLESS

Supermarkets are laid out to encourage you to buy more food – it's no coincidence the chocolate bars are by the checkout. To avoid impulse buys, plan your meals for the week and make a shopping list. But here's the most important part when you're cruising the aisles: stick to it! Your wallet will thank you as much as your waistline.

Sorry, there's no magic bullet. You gotta eat healthy and live healthy to be healthy and look healthy. End of story.

Morgan Spurlock

DON'T COUNT ON IT

Counting calories doesn't make you a healthy eater. People who tot up calories are often playing a game with themselves. If they eat unhealthy foods but stay within their calorie limit, they think they're winning. Not so! Focusing on calories rather than having a healthy, balanced diet can lead to low blood sugar levels, resulting in tiredness and erratic behaviour. To get out of the habit of calorie counting, focus on your body's feelings of hunger and being sated rather than numbers. Instead of opting for low-calorie meals, try to make nutritionally sensible choices. Vegetables, fruit and grains are always going to get the thumbs-up.

EAT FOODS YOUR FUTURE SELF WILL THANK YOU FOR.

PANDER TO YOUR PANCREAS

Your pancreas plays a crucial role in converting food into fuel for your body's cells. Its two main functions are to help with digestion and to regulate blood sugar. When you eat sugar, your pancreas releases insulin in order to process it, but when your sugar rush ends after a few minutes, your blood will still contain extra insulin. This results in a craving for more sweet foods. Curb these cravings before they even begin by eating plenty of fruit and sweet vegetables like butternut squash. Your pancreas will be pleased.

FORGET ME NOT

Do you sometimes forget to eat? Perhaps you've had a hectic day at work, you're stressed out or you simply haven't felt hungry. If you've missed breakfast and lunch, you may overcompensate come dinnertime by eating 'three meals in one', perhaps with quick-to-prepare and unhealthy food. Your body will be thinking, 'What the heck?' as it's not designed for this kind of inconsistent eating. Weight gain, low blood sugar levels and pancreatic problems could creep in. The brain won't be getting a regular dose of glucose, either, so your concentration could also be affected.

If you're frequently forgetting to eat, set a timer to remind you. You could also try planning ahead – if you know you'll be busy, busy, busy tomorrow, make your lunch the night before so you don't have to worry about it amid everything else on your plate, so to speak. A healthy snack in your bag (perhaps a portion of nuts) is also a good idea so you can refuel on the go.

IN MY FOOD WORLD,
THERE IS NO FEAR
OR GUILT. ONLY JOY
AND BALANCE. SO
NO INGREDIENT IS
EVER OFF-LIMITS.

Ellie Krieger

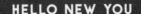

**Eat less of what
comes from a box
and more of what
comes from the earth.**

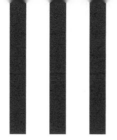

BROWN IS BETTER

If you want to shift a few pounds without too much effort, replace all white carbs with complex brown carbs, which are rich in fibre and nutrients. Instead of their white counterparts, eat brown bread, brown rice and brown pasta. Generally, the same portion will contain 20–40 per cent fewer calories.

SKIPPING MEALS IS A NO-NO

Never skip a meal if you're trying to lose weight. If you do, your blood sugar levels will plunge and you're more likely to crave a sugary fix. And don't bother with extreme diets – they never work long term and simply leave you hangry (hungry/angry).

EAT BETTER, NOT LESS.

CALL IN A PROFESSIONAL

If you're struggling to know where to start with healthy eating, don't be afraid to seek professional help. A nutritional therapist will evaluate your lifestyle habits, counsel you on food intolerance, give you a full-body composition check and devise a nutrition plan to help improve your health.

CHEW ON THIS

Overeating due to lack of portion control is a common problem that many of us face. Maybe you were 'programmed' as a child by your parents to clear your plate, or maybe you like the comforting feeling of being *super*-satisfied, or perhaps you just can't get enough of your mum's to-die-for cannelloni. Whatever the reason, overeating isn't healthy. Your stomach becomes overstuffed and the gastric acid struggles to break down the food, which leads to digestive issues such as diarrhoea, cramps, bloating and trapped wind. So, what can be done? Chew every mouthful until the food has turned into a liquid. As a result, your body will produce more amylase, the enzyme that helps with digestion. You'll lose weight, too, as chewing will help you feel fuller quicker.

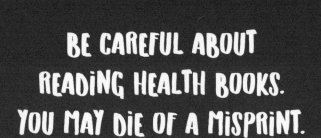

BE CAREFUL ABOUT
READING HEALTH BOOKS.
YOU MAY DIE OF A MISPRINT.

MARK TWAIN

PART 2
DRINK LESS

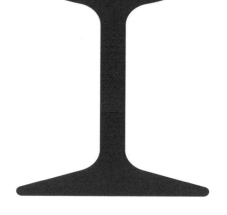

IT'S A GREAT ADVANTAGE NOT TO DRINK AMONG HARD-DRINKING PEOPLE.

F. SCOTT FITZGERALD

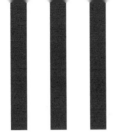

FOR GOOD REASON

Write down why you are deciding to drink less – perhaps you want to feel healthier, improve your relationships or you're simply sick of hangovers. Seeing the reasons in black and white will help to motivate you.

AND THE LIST GOES ON

Need reasons to drink less? Excessive consumption of alcohol can affect your health in both the short term and the long term. Here are a few effects:

Short-term effects

- Anxiety
- Blackouts
- Diarrhoea
- Disturbed sleep
- Impaired judgement, which can result in injuries or accidents
- Memory loss
- Shaking
- Skin conditions
- Stomach problems
- Stress
- Sweating
- Vomiting
- Weight gain

Long-term effects

- Brain damage
- Cancer
- Dementia
- Depression
- Heart disease
- High blood pressure
- Liver disease
- Mental health problems
- Osteoporosis
- Pancreatitis
- Reproductive problems
- Stomach ulcers
- Stroke

**Positive anything
is better than
negative nothing.**

Elbert Hubbard

SUPPORT ACT

Tell your family and friends that you've decided to cut back your drinking. They can offer you support and will know not to pour you another when your glass is empty.

ALCOHOL IS NOT THE ANSWER – IT JUST MAKES YOU FORGET THE QUESTION.

SKIN DEEP

Every time you drink, your body gets dehydrated, and this has a huge impact on your skin. It's deprived of the vital nutrients and vitamins it needs to stay healthy, so can become dull and grey. Not a good look! Luckily, skin reacts quickly to change, so it can return to normal after only a couple of days of cutting back on booze. However, over time, heavy drinking can have long-lasting, harmful effects on your skin. Rosacea, a skin disorder that starts with a tendency to blush profusely and can lead to permanent redness in the face, or even facial disfigurement, has been linked to alcohol. Research found that those who drank alcohol had an increased risk of rosacea compared to those who didn't drink, and that this risk increased the more they drank.

DOING THE ROUNDS

You'll probably drink – and spend –
more if you get involved in buying rounds
in a bar as you'll be trying to keep up
with the fastest drinker in the group.
Give rounds a miss, or just do smaller
rounds with a couple of friends.

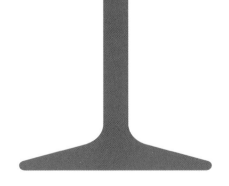

THAT'S ALL DRUGS
AND ALCOHOL DO;
THEY CUT OFF YOUR
EMOTIONS IN THE END.

RINGO STARR

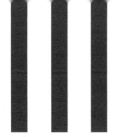

THE MEASURE
OF THINGS

Buy an alcohol measure so you know how much you're drinking when pouring your own drinks at home. Also, don't keep refilling your wine glass before you finish what's in there – you'll only drink more that way.

HANDLE THE PRESSURE

Drinking to excess can have a negative impact on your blood pressure. High blood pressure can lead to a heart attack or stroke. To reduce the risks, it's a good idea to drink sensibly, eat well and exercise regularly.

A WEIGHTY ISSUE

Alcohol can make you gain weight – and not just because a glass of wine contains the same calories as four cookies while a pint of beer is as calorific as a large slice of pizza. Research has also shown that drinking alcohol gives you the munchies because the neurons in your brain that provoke hunger are activated by alcohol. That's why, come 2 a.m., you may often find yourself in the kebab shop. And just as the calories from alcohol are 'empty calories' – they have no nutritional value – the fast food you consume contains very little in the way of nutrients.

SWITCH UP
YOUR VENUES

Limit the time you spend in bars and pubs. Instead, meet people in coffee shops, restaurants or even an alcohol-free bar (yes, they do exist). And if you're watching a sporting event, invite friends over to yours – you'll almost certainly drink less than you would at a bar surrounded by drunk fans.

I DRINK TOO MUCH.
THE LAST TIME I GAVE
A URINE SAMPLE IT
HAD AN OLIVE IN IT.

Rodney Dangerfield

LESS DRINKING, MORE THINKING.

REMOVE TEMPTATION

Don't keep alcohol in your house – get rid
of bottles of spirits, avoid stocking up on
wine… and that sticky bottle of something
at the back of your cupboard? Trash it!
If it's not there, you can't drink it.

EXERCISE SOME CONTROL

Alcohol and exercise are not a good combination. It's common sense not to hit the gym after a couple of drinks. Not only will you become more dehydrated than you usually would, your energy levels, coordination, reactions and concentration will also be impaired, leading to a lacklustre – and possibly dangerous – workout. Similarly, consuming alcohol the night before will have a negative impact on your workout performance the next day. You'll feel tired more quickly because your body won't be able to eliminate the lactic acid you produce when you exercise, plus your power and strength will be compromised. Not to mention the fact that a hangover can cause dehydration, a headache, sickness and the shakes.

SAY NO TO A NIGHTCAP

Drinking alcohol near bedtime may help you get to sleep initially but will prevent you from reaching a deep sleep. You're also more likely to wake early. Stop drinking two or three hours before you go to bed, and drink one glass of water for every glass of alcohol to dodge dehydration and inspire some decent shut-eye.

DON'T DRINK TO GET DRUNK.

FIND ALTERNATIVES

Do you use booze as a crutch, drinking
when you're lonely, angry or worried?
Try to find new, healthy ways to cope
when you feel like reaching for a drink.
Perhaps go for a run, call a friend
or listen to your favourite song
to lift your spirits.

**The rule is simple:
be sober and temperate,
and you will be healthy.**

Benjamin Franklin

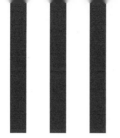

UNDER THE WEATHER

Too much alcohol can interfere with your immune system, meaning you're more likely to get ill. Start drinking less and you'll soon have more energy, and feel less sluggish and tired.

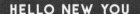

You don't need
alcohol to have fun.

FEELING BLUE

Alcohol affects your mental health. The neurotransmitters in our brains are altered by alcohol and this can influence our feelings, thoughts and actions. Alcohol is a depressant, so anxiety, depression and stress can all be heightened by drinking too much. On one end of the scale, you may get 'beer fear' after a night out ('Oh no, did I *really* do/say/dance on that?'). On the more serious end of the scale, alcohol is often linked to self-harm and suicide. If you regularly drink heavily, the levels of serotonin in your brain – a chemical that helps to balance your mood – will be lowered, which may lead to feelings of depression.

DRINKING RESPONSIBLY DOES NOT MEAN NOT SPILLING IT.

WORK IT

Don't let alcohol stand in the way of
your professional success. Drinking too
much at lunch or the night before can
affect your concentration at work,
hindering your performance.
Drink less to work smarter.

FEWER SIPS FOR SMOOTHER SKIN

Alcohol can exacerbate cellulite. The toxins it contains may contribute to the build-up of unsightly orange-peel skin. Booze also encourages fluid retention and increases fatty deposits in areas such as your thighs, stomach, arms and bottom.

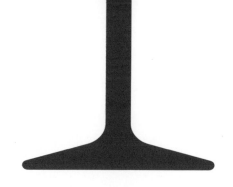

IF ONE OVERSTEPS
THE BOUNDS OF
MODERATION, THE
GREATEST PLEASURES
CEASE TO PLEASE.

EPICTETUS

LIFE IS BETTER SOBER.

FOOD FOR THOUGHT

Once you've opened a bottle of wine, consider cooking with the leftovers rather than drinking it. Freeze leftover wine in an ice-cube tray to use in cooking as and when you need it. You don't have to drink every drop.

EXCUSE ME

Many people give themselves 'permission' to get drunk with one excuse or another. If you find yourself justifying your drinking with any of these 'reasons', it could be time to cut back:

'It's the weekend'

That 'Friday feeling' of not having to get up for work in the morning can cause some people to get carried away with their alcohol consumption. If you don't want a hangover to ruin your time off, alternate your alcoholic drinks with soft ones or water.

'I need Dutch courage'

Do you get nervous in social situations so you drink to lower your inhibitions? If so, try going to places where there's more on offer than alcohol. Seeing a band, going to the theatre or watching a film at the cinema will mean there's less pressure to drink than if you're simply sat in a bar.

'I've had a bad day'

Drinking to deal with stress is common but, as alcohol is a depressant, it can often make things worse. Instead of boozing after a tough day at work, why not go for a run? Exercise can help to relax your body and mind.

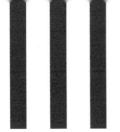

LET UP ON YOUR LIVER

If you drink regularly, your body – your liver in particular – will begin to build up a tolerance to alcohol and you'll need to drink more and more to obtain the same 'buzz'. Give your body a break and have some alcohol-free days. How about teetotal Tuesdays? Or mocktail Mondays?

AVOID USING
CIGARETTES.
ALCOHOL. AND DRUGS
AS ALTERNATIVES
TO BEING AN
INTERESTING PERSON.

Marilyn vos Savant

FROM SIZZLE TO FIZZLE

Drinking alcohol to excess can affect your sex life. For men, in the short term, 'brewer's droop' (the inability to maintain an erection) can put a dampener on things; in the long term, full-on impotence may occur. Alcohol can also affect fertility in both men and women. So lay off the booze before you hit the bedroom – if nothing else, sober sex is more of a thrill for your senses and your partner.

DON'T DRINK TO DROWN YOUR SORROWS. SORROWS KNOW HOW TO SWIM.

THIRST THINGS FIRST

When you're thirsty, especially on a night out, it's tempting to opt for a bigger drink - a large glass of wine rather than a small one. **But you shouldn't slake your thirst with alcohol, as you'll just drink more, spend more and the booze will leave you dehydrated in the long run. Instead, order a large glass of water alongside your drink. Start with a big gulp of that to quench your initial thirst, then alternate sips of alcohol and sips of water.**

DON'T WORRY, BE APPY

Download an app that can help you keep track of your drinking. There are loads to choose from, and they will do everything from calculating the units and calories you consume, to reviewing your drinking habits over time, plus offering support, guidance and motivation. Alternatively, you could use a journal to keep track of everything.

NOT HAVING ALCOHOL
HAS KEPT THE WEIGHT
OFF AROUND MY
WAIST: MY SKIN FEELS
SO MUCH BETTER.
AND I AM SLEEPING
REALLY WELL.

Marie Helvin

NEVER DRINK ON AN EMPTY STOMACH. NUFF SAID.

HOW LOW CAN YOU GO?

Choose drinks with a low or reduced alcohol content. 'Low-alcohol drinks' refer to beverages that have an alcoholic strength by volume (ABV) of between 0.5 and 1.2 per cent. 'Reduced-alcohol drinks' have an alcohol content lower than the average strength of a particular drink. Assuming you still consume the same number of drinks, going for these options can help you to stay within recommended drinking guidelines. This will have a positive impact on your health. In the immediate future, you'll get a better night's sleep, avoid a hangover and be more productive the following day. Further down the line, reducing the number of units you drink will decrease your risk of mental health problems, cancer, heart disease and high blood pressure.

Substituting your regular tipple with one lower in alcohol is an easy and sustainable approach to cutting down your drinking. So, if you go for a glass of wine after work, you will more than halve the number of units you drink by swapping the usual 12–14 per cent to a 5.5 per cent one. Over time, this will reduce the negative health effects of alcohol dramatically.

KICK THE HABIT

Drinking is often done out of habit. For example, you may get home from work, open the fridge and get yourself a beer, or pour yourself a large glass of wine every night with dinner. To cut back, try to reset these habits by opting for a different beverage in these scenarios. Try to find a non-alcoholic drink that will still be a treat – perhaps a flavoured pressé or a zingy ginger ale.

EATING IS NOT CHEATING

Drunkorexia is a phenomenon mainly affecting young women who are concerned with gaining weight through alcohol and so skip meals to save calories. Often they do this with the intention of binge drinking, with the motto 'eating's cheating' in their minds. This is, obviously, not a great way to stay healthy. In the short term, starving yourself in order to overindulge in drink can lead to vomiting, passing out and alcohol poisoning. Doing this on a regular basis could seriously damage your liver and heart. As alcohol contains no nutrients, you're also more likely to be missing out on vital vitamins and minerals in the food that you're not eating. Eating healthily before or during drinking is a much better idea and, for those conscious of calories, it's better to cut back on alcohol rather than food.

WINE IS A
TURNCOAT;
FIRST, A FRIEND;
THEN, A DECEIVER;
THEN, AN ENEMY.

TRADITIONAL SAYING

PLAY SWAPSIES

Opt for the non-alcoholic equivalent of your tipple of choice. These days, you can find non-alcoholic beer, wine and even spirits. There are countless mocktails that taste just as delicious as their alcoholic counterparts. The best thing? No hangover.

If one is never enough, have none.

TREAT YOURSELF FOR BEING TEETOTAL

A bottle of wine here, a round in the pub there... The amount you spend on booze can quickly add up. Each time you choose not to have a drink, put aside the money you would have spent. Then at the end of the month use it to treat yourself to something that will give you more lasting pleasure and value than booze, and without the negative side-effects.

MIX THINGS UP

Turn your white wine into a spritzer, using
lemonade or soda water as a mixer. Or get your
Spanish on and whip up some calimocho, which
is red wine with cola. If you use half a small
glass of wine (about 60 ml/2 fl oz), there will be
less than one unit of alcohol in each glass.

LIFE'S TOO SHORT TO WASTE ON HANGOVERS.

IGNORANCE IS A LOT LIKE ALCOHOL: THE MORE YOU HAVE OF IT, THE LESS YOU ARE ABLE TO SEE ITS EFFECT ON YOU.

JAY M. BYLSMA

SEEING STARS

Take some inspiration from these teetotal celebrities:

- **Jennifer Lopez**, aka J-Lo, says 'J-No' to drinking. The singer and actress says, 'I think that ruins your skin.'

- Actor **Gerard Butler** avoids alcohol these days, saying: 'I did a full life's worth of drinking between 14 and 27.'

- Model **Tyra Banks** tried alcohol when she was 12 and decided never to drink again.

- Country singer **Tim McGraw** quit drinking in 2008 after his wife, Faith Hill, warned him that alcohol was taking over his life.

- *Sex and the City* actresses **Kim Cattrall** and **Kristin Davis** may have made the cosmopolitan cocktail famous but neither of them actually drink.

- Actress and singer **Jennifer Hudson** says she's never had a drink in her life.

- *Friends* actor **Matthew Perry** struggled with alcoholism while he was filming the show but has since decided to go sober.

- Actress **Natalie Portman** has embraced the teetotal lifestyle.

- DJ **Calvin Harris** says that since giving up alcohol, his live shows are 'a million times better'.

- *Gossip Girl* star **Blake Lively** says that she has no desire to drink.

PART 3
EXERCISE MORE

EXERCISE TO
STIMULATE, NOT
TO ANNIHILATE.
THE WORLD WASN'T
FORMED IN A DAY, AND
NEITHER WERE WE.
SET SMALL GOALS AND
BUILD UPON THEM.

Lee Haney

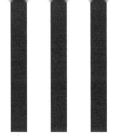

QUESTION YOURSELF

Ask yourself what you want to achieve from your exercise regime. Do you want to lose weight? Feel healthier? Increase your fitness? Then ask yourself why. Perhaps you want to fit into your wedding outfit, be happier or complete a half-marathon. When you know why something is important to you, your motivation will increase.

FEELING IT

To maximize performance, match your workout to your mood.

If you're **STRESSED**, try yoga. Refocusing your mind and breathing deeply will do you the world of good. Yoga releases muscle tension, especially in the back, neck and shoulders, which may be tight after a stressful day.

If you're **HAPPY**, try Zumba. Zumba involves both dance and aerobics, and is very sociable. Also, when you're in good spirits, you're open to new experiences, so try something new like hip-hop dance, hula hooping or even a trapeze class.

If you're **ANGRY**, try kickboxing. Hitting the you-know-what out of a punchbag will relieve your rage and release endorphins, the 'happy hormones'. Channel the adrenaline that anger produces to really crush your workout.

If you're **ENERGIZED**, try a cardio workout like spinning or circuit training. They're demanding and you often have to push through the pain barrier mid-workout, so you've got to be in the right frame of mind.

If you're **SAD**, try exercising outdoors. Fresh air, natural light, the sights, sounds and smells of nature – an outside workout will boost your mood more than exercising in a sweaty gym. Try running, cycling or walking in your local park and your frown will soon be turned upside down.

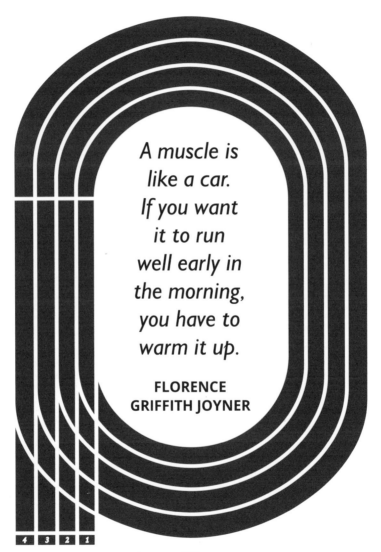

A muscle is like a car. If you want it to run well early in the morning, you have to warm it up.

FLORENCE GRIFFITH JOYNER

STRETCHING:
THE TRUTH

It's important to stretch your muscles before you exercise, right? Wrong! Never stretch your muscles when they're cold. If you do, you could actually weaken them and make your performance slower. Always stretch after you've exercised – either after your warm-up (for example, a gentle jog, marching on the spot or skipping for a few minutes) or at the end of your workout.

EXERCISE IS NATURE'S ANTIDEPRESSANT.

MORNING MOTIVATION

Get your day off to a blood-pumping start. As your day progresses, and other things crop up, exercise can often be downgraded as an 'I'll do it later/tomorrow' activity. But if you prioritize a workout in the morning, other pressures can't interfere and you'll find it easier to stick to your routine. Getting your heart rate up will also release feel-good endorphins, which will set you on a positive path for the rest of the day. Why not kill three birds with one stone and run/cycle/walk to work? You'll get fit, get to work and save money. Win-win-win!

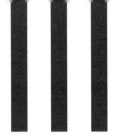

WE CAN WORK IT OUT

It's important to always include a warm-up and a cooldown into each workout, but what you do in-between can vary wildly. Alternate these different types of workouts to keep things interesting:

- A cardio/aerobic workout – running, bike-riding, skipping, boxing, rowing
- Resistance/strength-building exercises – using resistance bands, lifting weights
- Flexibility moves – stretching, yoga, Pilates

NOTHING LIFTS ME
OUT OF A BAD MOOD
BETTER THAN A HARD
WORKOUT ON MY
TREADMILL. IT NEVER
FAILS. EXERCISE
IS NOTHING SHORT
OF A MIRACLE.

Cher

SLOW AND STEADY
WINS THE RACE

It's great when motivation strikes, but one of the biggest mistakes often made with exercise is to begin too fast, only to quickly fatigue. Then we think that we've failed and give up. Keep it slow and increase things steadily to build your stamina and confidence.

BODY, YOU'LL THANK ME LATER.

MAKE A SPLASH

Swimming is a great all-round exercise for the entire body. It's ideal for pregnant women and those who can't do weight-bearing exercise as the water takes stress off the joints. Work up to a good swim workout. Start by doing one session a week, swimming for about 10-20 minutes. Try to swim continuously but don't worry if you need to rest every so often. When you can do this comfortably, try interval swimming, where you swim one length at an easy pace, then one at a harder pace. Then one easy, followed by two harder. Then three… four… you get the idea. Increase the time you spend swimming, the number of lengths and the number of sessions per week. Vary your routine to include a variety of strokes – front crawl, breaststroke, backstroke and butterfly – which will strengthen different areas of your body.

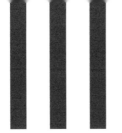

STOP OR DROP

No pain, no gain? No! Whatever exercise you're doing, you should either stop or slow down if you're experiencing pain, dizziness or nausea. And don't ignore your niggles – you could end up with a permanent injury. Take a moment, rest if needed and figure out the reason for your twinges. If the pain persists, see your doctor.

JOGGING IS VERY
BENEFICIAL. IT'S GOOD
FOR YOUR LEGS AND
YOUR FEET. IT'S ALSO
VERY GOOD FOR THE
GROUND. IT MAKES
IT FEEL NEEDED.

Charles M. Schulz

BREATHE EASY

It's important to wear the right kit. Trainers that have mesh incorporated into their design will allow your feet to breathe and will keep your feet cool and comfortable. Plus, as your feet are sweating less, your trainers won't get so smelly. Be sure to wear lightweight clothing to train in to avoid profuse sweating – there's a lot of sports gear on the market these days that will wick perspiration away from your skin.

UP FOR THE CHALLENGE

To maintain your motivation, sign up for a physical challenge – perhaps a 10k run, a long swim or a demanding bike ride. As you work towards your goal, you'll stay focused on your training and will also make healthier lifestyle choices. For added motivation, enter a sponsored event in support of a charity.

BE A POSER

Yoga is a great workout for people of all fitness levels. It focuses on flexibility, strength, balance and breathing to enhance physical and mental well-being. Each yoga pose can bring different benefits. There are plenty of online videos and tutorials showing you how to do them. Try out these poses:

Downward Dog sends fresh oxygen and blood to your spine, which will rejuvenate the body. It will boost your core strength, while leaving you less tense and more relaxed.

Cobra Pose stretches the muscles on the front of your torso, while strengthening your arms and shoulders. It's particularly valuable for people who spend a lot of time sitting down as this can make the muscles at the front of your body tight.

The **Bridge** is great for opening your front hip joints, while strengthening your spine, opening your chest and improving your spinal flexibility. It also stimulates your thyroid, which can regulate metabolism and boost energy.

Child Pose is a resting pose and relieves neck, back and hip tension. It's helpful to return to this pose frequently as it is one of the most calming, restorative poses.

The **Crow** strengthens your upper back, wrists, forearms and abs, while also stretching the hamstrings. It can also help to decrease heartburn. Good balance is vital for this pose.

PUT SOME MUSCLE INTO IT

If you want to build muscle and increase your metabolism, get into sprint training, which involves sprinting for a short burst (perhaps 30 seconds to a minute), then walking for a couple of minutes, followed by another sprint – then repeating. This will stimulate human growth hormone (HGH), helping you burn fat and build muscle. Strength training – perhaps using resistance bands or dumbbells – is also a good plan.

LOOK IN THE MIRROR. THAT'S YOUR COMPETITION.

TIMING IS EVERYTHING

Exercising too close to bedtime can affect the production of melatonin, the hormone that aids sleep. To ensure your body is in 'sleep mode' rather than 'active mode', exercise at least three hours before lights out. Working out in the late afternoon or early evening is said to be most beneficial for a good night's sleep.

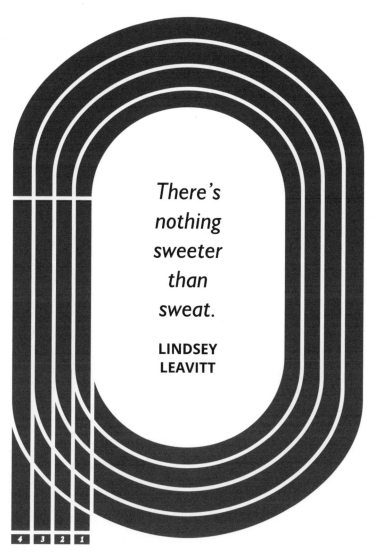

There's nothing sweeter than sweat.

LINDSEY LEAVITT

Motivation comes and goes. The key is learning how to build habits.

A HOME WIN

Hate gyms or can't afford a membership?
Work out at home! Use equipment that will
keep things interesting and challenging – like
an exercise ball, skipping rope or resistance
bands. You could set up a mini circuit class
and invite friends round to join in.

SQUAT'S THE DEAL?

Squats do more than strengthen your legs. They also: increase the entire body's strength and muscle; burn fat; improve circulation; reduce cellulite; increase flexibility; improve posture; build core strength; tone your abs, legs and bottom; help you maintain mobility and balance; and make household tasks like cleaning, gardening, shopping and decorating easier!

The difficulty of a squat can vary. Sitting down on a chair is a simple squat and a good place to start. As you sit down, then stand up again from a chair, keep your weight central and don't use your arms to assist you. Do this for two sets of 10 repetitions. When you're ready to ramp up your squats, stand with your feet shoulder-width apart, toes forward. Place your hands on your thighs, look up and lift your chest high. Bend your knees, moving your weight onto your heels, and sit back. Keeping the head and chest up, slide your hands down your thighs and beyond, ending when your elbows reach your knees (ensure your knees don't stick out further than your toes). Hold for five seconds. Begin to stand up, pressing through your heels, and straighten out your hips until you're in the position you started in. Repeat 15 to 20 times, for two or three sets. Be sure to keep your back straight to avoid injury. It's a good idea to do squats in front of a mirror so you can see if the position of your body looks right.

YOU HAVE A CHOICE.
YOU CAN EITHER
THROW IN THE
TOWEL OR USE IT
TO WIPE THE SWEAT
FROM YOUR FACE.

MOVE MORE

Inconvenience yourself. Take the stairs instead of the elevator, park further away than you had planned, walk to the next bus stop, get off the sofa to change the channel. Adding incidental exercise into your daily routine may do more good than you realize.

PHYSICAL FITNESS
IS NOT ONLY ONE OF
THE MOST IMPORTANT
KEYS TO A HEALTHY
BODY. IT IS THE
BASIS OF DYNAMIC
AND CREATIVE
INTELLECTUAL
ACTIVITY.

John F. Kennedy

FIND A FITNESS FRIEND

Having an exercise buddy is a great motivation to keep you on track. You'll spur each other on, and encourage each other to actually turn up. Sometimes, it's all-too-tempting to put a workout off until tomorrow (which never comes), but if you've committed to your friend, you won't want to let them down.

TIRED? OUT OF BREATH? SWEATY? GOOD... IT'S WORKING.

BUST A GROOVE

Depending on how much you weigh, dancing for just 15 minutes can burn up to 100 calories. So whether you're taking a dance class or shimmying around your living room, throwing shapes will certainly get your heart going.

STRESS LESS

Work! Kids! Bills! Chores! *Arrgh!* Stress is the worst, and has a negative impact on us physically and emotionally. It can deplete your immune system and contribute to headaches, heart problems, high blood pressure, skin conditions, diabetes, insomnia, arthritis, anxiety and depression. It will also slow down your body's metabolism, leading to poor digestion. On top of all this, it will increase your levels of the stress hormone cortisol, which can ultimately increase body fat. Combat this by zenning out with Pilates, yoga and meditation. Try to do at least 10 minutes of deep diaphragmatic breaths a day. Place one hand on your belly and one on your chest, then feel both lift and deflate as you inhale and exhale. Focusing on deep breathing encourages your body to burn fat, keeps you calm and reduces stress. Aaaaand... breathe...

MAKE TIME

Staying fit makes you more productive. Keep this in mind if you're slammed at work and simply *can't* find the time to exercise. Remember that if you make time for a workout, you'll ultimately get more done as your energy levels will be boosted, as will your ability to concentrate.

Fitness is not about being better than someone else – it's about being better than you used to be.

Anonymous

THE ONLY BAD WORKOUT IS THE ONE THAT DIDN'T HAPPEN.

WALKING BACK
TO HAPPINESS

Walking is a fantastic way to stay healthy and lose weight. Nordic walking is even better! Because you're holding poles, you will be using the muscles in your arms, shoulders and torso, meaning an all-body workout that burns 20 per cent more calories than regular walking.

HIT IT

As well as being a fun sport to play, tennis can have a positive impact on your mind, body and life in general. Here are a few reasons to pick up a racket:

- Tennis is a fantastic all-over body workout. You'll run, jump, reach, swing, lunge, sprint and pivot. You'll require flexibility, balance, strength, speed, coordination, stamina and mobility, while using a lot of muscle groups and joints. It's also a great way to improve your bone strength and density.

- Creativity is key in tennis as a game/set/match requires tactical thinking and planning. Every rally is different, so tennis can be extremely mentally stimulating. The brain is engaged as much as the body. Studies have shown that exercise which demands a lot of thinking improves memory, the ability to learn, social skills, behaviour and, of course, reaction times. Optimism and self-esteem are also bolstered.

- Hand–eye coordination is vital in tennis – and in life, for tasks such as writing and painting. Spatial awareness, visual sharpness and fine motor skills are also essential both on the court and in everyday life.

YOU'LL GET THERE

Some sessions will go better than others. That's OK – you're not a robot! Every session you complete will get you closer to your goals. The important thing is to keep going.

THE MIND IS THE MOST
IMPORTANT PART
OF ACHIEVING ANY
FITNESS GOAL. MENTAL
CHANGE ALWAYS
COMES BEFORE
PHYSICAL CHANGE.

Matt McGorry

SWEAT IT OUT

If you're doing it right, exercise will likely make you sweat. Sweating is a great way to detoxify, and it will also help you feel less bloated as sweat contains a lot of sodium, as well as other electrolytes. If you have an all-out sweat-fest, it might be an idea to take an electrolyte tablet after your workout to replenish the minerals you lose. You should also eat – preferably carbs – 30 minutes after you exercise in order to refuel and help your muscles to recover. A banana is ideal: it's rich in potassium, magnesium and fast-working carbohydrates. And remember to stay hydrated with plenty of water.

MORE SWEAT NOW, LESS JIGGLE LATER.

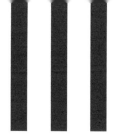

LISTEN UP

If you get bored while you're training, listen to a podcast, a feel-good playlist you've compiled or an audiobook to keep you entertained and motivated to punch through the monotony.

THE LONG RUN

Running is a mind game. No matter how experienced you are, or how far you're running, your mind will always be your biggest challenge. Try alternating these two techniques during a run and you may just be able to go that extra mile:

- **Associate.** Be in the moment and don't think about the finish line. Take in the environment and sense how your body is feeling. This is a great technique to acknowledge where you are in your run and to tune in to your body so that you can change the intensity or pace according to your plan.

- **Dissociate.** Travel in your mind. Think about anything but the running you're doing and you'll find you feel less tired (or less bored). Go through a shopping list, your to-do list, plan your next holiday... Also, imagine you're running on a deserted beach or a beautiful mountain trail – anything that lets your mind go somewhere else and stops you from looking at your watch, feeling how tired you are or thinking about how far you have left to go.

*Practice puts
brains in
your muscles.*

SAM SNEAD

PATIENCE IS A VIRTUE

You want a six-pack and you want it yesterday! It's important to manage your expectations – don't expect miracles after one workout. Instead, keep chipping away, gaining momentum as you go. Expecting too much too soon will lead to demotivation, so be patient. Results will happen.

NO MATTER HOW SLOW YOU GO, YOU ARE STILL LAPPING EVERYONE ON THE SOFA.

FEEL IT IN YOUR BONES

As we age, the health of our bones begins to decline, which can ultimately lead to them becoming brittle. Our spine and lower-body bones support our weight, so are obviously very important. To keep bones stronger for longer, and build bone density, choose weight-bearing exercises like aerobics, resistance training and walking.

We do not stop exercising because we grow old... we grow old because we stop exercising.

Kenneth H. Cooper

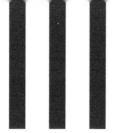

FIND YOUR FIT

Do exercise you love. Don't spend hours pounding it out on a treadmill if you don't enjoy it. Find something that you'll look forward to doing. Try lots of different things – synchronized swimming, trampolining, ballet, aerial yoga or simply power walking in the park – until you find the right fit for you.

BE STRONGER THAN YOUR EXCUSES.

DIFFERENT STROKES FOR DIFFERENT FOLKS

Sometimes, the wrong type of exercise can be just as bad as doing none at all. We are all different and not everyone's bodies are capable of the same things. Take running, for example: if you're not built for it, it can be damaging to your hips and knees. And yoga? Some of us just aren't meant to be that flexible. Exercise should never cause you extended discomfort. Trying a new activity often causes DOMS (delayed onset muscle soreness), which occurs as you use muscle groups in ways you haven't for some time, but this should never last for more than three days. Ultimately, pushing ourselves is positive but it should never be harmful to our bodies. If you've tried something and it's not for you, try something different.

CONCLUSION

So, there you have it – a guide to eating better, drinking less and exercising more. Life is all about choices, and hopefully you will choose to incorporate these tips, nuggets of advice and words of inspiration into your everyday life. Don't let them get lost among your daily frazzled rush, endless to-do lists and groaning inbox. Instead, embrace them to bring further joy into your life, amid silliness with friends, belly laughs and random acts of kindness.

As with any lifestyle change, if you have any concerns, please speak to a medical professional. They will be able to offer guidance as to the best course of action, should you need an extra helping hand. The first step to change is always the hardest, but you won't regret it. If you wake every morning with determination, you'll go to bed at night with satisfaction. So... eat well, move daily, hydrate often, sleep lots, love your body, repeat for life.

Goodbye excuses. Goodbye sluggish body. Goodbye negative mindset.

Hello New You.

Have you enjoyed this book?
If so, why not write a review on your favourite website?

If you're interested in finding out more about our books,
find us on Facebook at **Summersdale Publishers** and
follow us on Twitter at **@Summersdale**.

Thanks very much for buying this Summersdale book.

www.summersdale.com